THE CAT
APPOINTMENT

Fiction for Seniors

seniorality

chapter 1
Something To Do

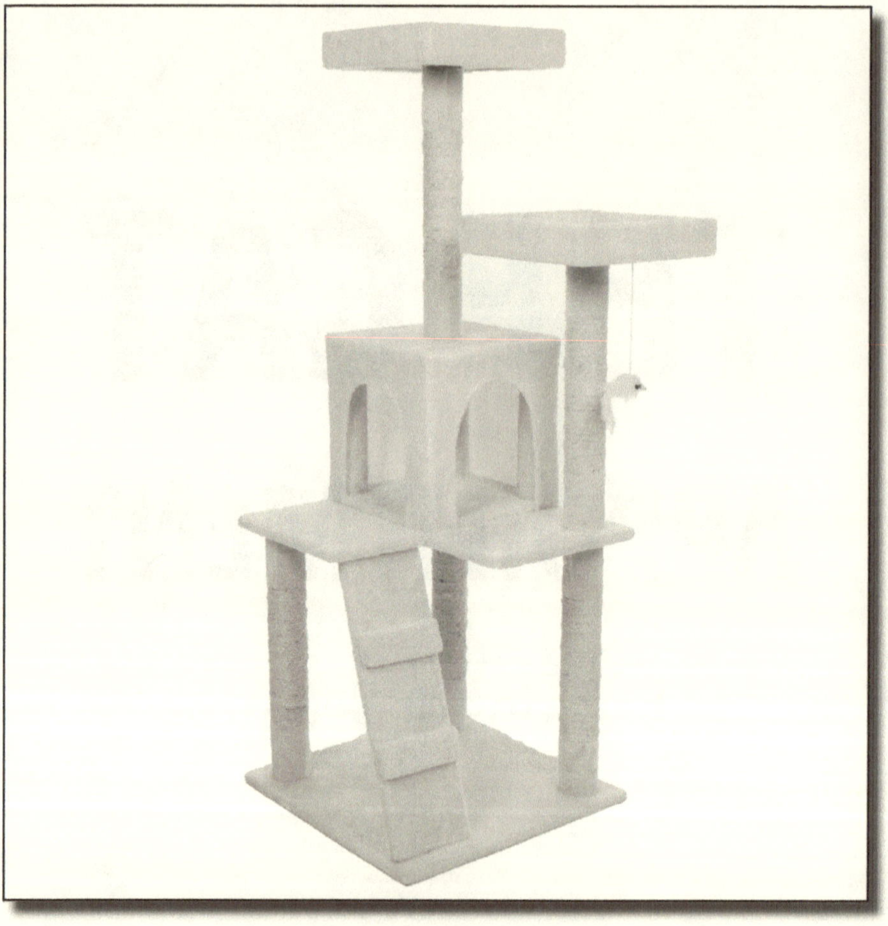

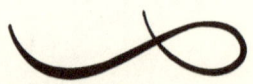

FROM THE MOMENT I woke up, I knew I had to do something this morning.

I started with my stretches while I was under my blanket. I wiggled my fingers and toes. Next, I pointed and relaxed my feet.

After that, I would bend my knees and then straighten them out. It was so much easier to stretch a little bit at a time.

It was time to get out of bed. I sat up and slowly got out from under my soft blanket. I had my slippers on my feet right away because I could feel the chill on the floor. The soft, fuzzy shoes also made it comfortable to take each step away from my bedroom and around my house.

I put my hands over my head and stretched some more. This was my favorite moment as

I woke up. But I still had more to do this morning. When my body was ready, I stood up and left my bedroom.

I walked down the hallway and said hello to each face on the wall. Some of the photos were black and white even though I lived that life in color. Other pictures were of children who do not look so little anymore.

When I looked in my living room, I first saw my favorite chair. The red covering on the chair was worn in the seat and in the arms. Those spots were also the softest parts of the chair. I sit in that chair to read, listen to music, or watch TV.

Since I just woke up, I was not tired or ready to relax. My day was just beginning.

I also saw a tower near the bookshelf by the far wall. The tower almost looked like an old tree in winter. It was covered in brown carpet and stood almost as tall as me. It looked like it could hold items on it like picture frames or glass. It was empty.

The door to the laundry room was open. Today I would check to make sure I have enough socks in my drawers. I go through a lot of socks when the days get cooler in the fall. Sometimes they get so worn out that I get a hole by the toes or under the heel. My feet get cold when that happens.

In between the washing machine and dryer, there was a gray box with a cover over it. It looked like a plastic cave that was perfect for hiding.

There was a little bit of something in front of the opening. It looked like sand or pebbles. I needed to sweep that up later before it got all over the room.

Nothing else in the room caught my attention, so I continued my walk to the kitchen. I saw the coffee maker on the counter. I was ready for a warm mug of coffee this morning.

The mug was already in the machine. It was one of those one-cup makers that my grandkids got me last year. I thought it would be too hard to use, but it was perfect for me. All I had to do was put the package of coffee into the top of the machine and press the power button.

I opened the refrigerator to get out the milk. My box of cereal and bowl were already on the table. I took the milk and coffee to the table and sat down for breakfast.

My foot kicked something under the table. I looked down to see a mouse, but I knew it was not a real one. Not only was it too small to be a real mouse, but it also made a squeaking noise like toys do when they are squeezed.

I did not want to step on that toy again. I kicked the toy mouse toy out of the way and made sure it was not under where my foot would go again. It squeaked as it crossed the kitchen floor.

The moment that the mouse squeaked, there was a bell ringing from the laundry room. A cat with golden fur walked into the kitchen. The bell on his collar jingled with every step.

When it saw the mouse toy on the kitchen floor, it jumped on the toy. It rolled on its back and held on to the toy. The toy squeaked as it was squeezed between two paws.

"Good morning," I said to the cat.

"Meow," it said back to me. It continued to play with its mouse toy.

I looked next to the pantry and saw the dishes on the floor. One was for food and one was for water. The name Toby was written in white on the front of the blue dish.

Now I knew what I had to do this morning.

chapter 2
Feeding Toby

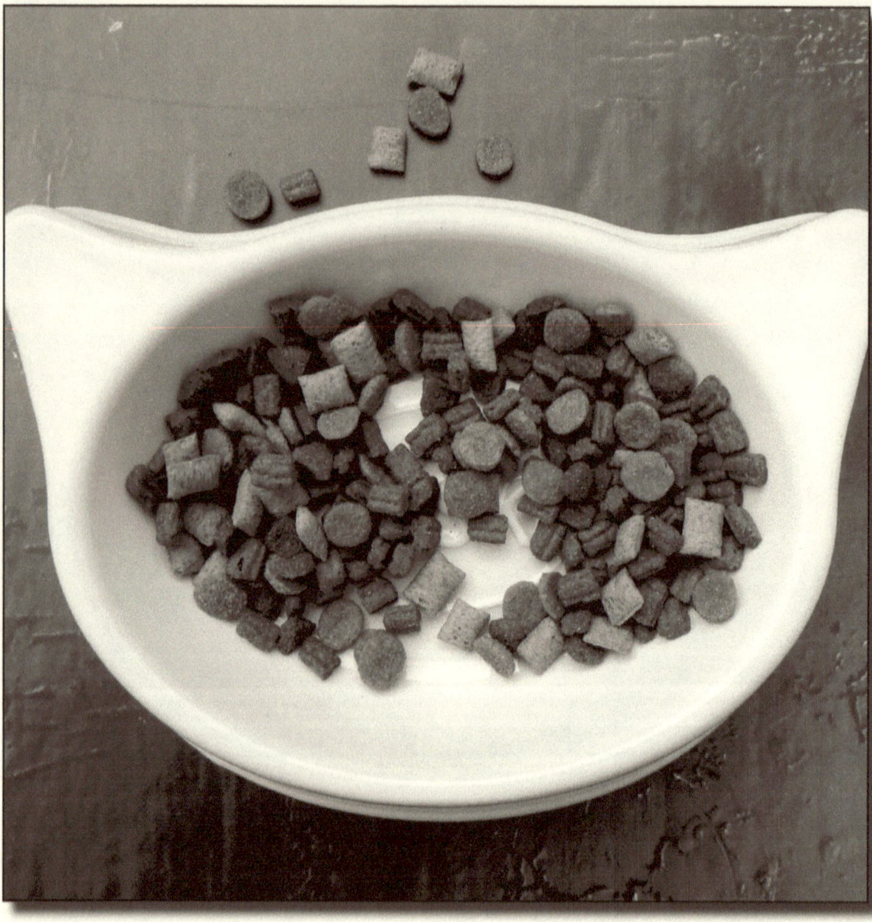

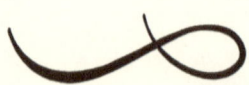

I WATCHED my cat, Toby, play some more on the kitchen floor while I ate my cereal and milk. I started to think about the many the cats I'd had in my life.

We had many cats in our family. My mom loved cats, so we always had one or two as I was growing up. After I got married, we continued to have cats as part of the family.

Some of the cats were very loving and wanted to be on our laps. They were by our feet when we were cooking. A few cats liked to be in our home, but they preferred to take naps by the window or be alone.

Toby was the kind of cat that was playful in his own slow way. He liked to do things but was not in a rush to do it. He was amusing to watch as he played with his toys or the sunlight on the floor.

Toby was also an agreeable cat. He did not ignore me, but he also did not need my attention all the time. We got along very well for these reasons.

I got up from the table and put the cereal bowl in the sink. Next, I put the milk back in the refrigerator. Toby noticed that I was done with my breakfast. He started meowing.

"Let me look in your bowl and see what you need," I told Toby.

The one with his name on it was the food dish. There were a few pieces of dry bits in it. The other one was the water bowl. There was still water on the bottom, but some of the food got into it.

I picked up the water bowl and took it to the sink. I rinsed the food out and added fresh water to the bowl. I only filled it halfway. That made it easier for me to carry it back to his food area without spilling any on the way there.

Once I placed the water in its spot, I picked up the food dish and placed it on the counter. I stopped for a moment to think about what I should feed Toby.

I remembered that the bag of cat food was in the pantry. It was very heavy so I must keep it in one place where I don't have to lift it. I took the bowl to the pantry, opened the tall bag, and used the scoop inside to fill the bowl enough for breakfast. One small scoop was enough for his morning meal.

I took the bowl back to the counter and looked in the cabinet above. There I found some cans with pictures of cats on it. I read the labels to see what we had.

"It looks like tender turkey pate today," I told Toby. The cat agreed with me and said, "Meow".

The lid had a pull tab on it. Sometimes those tabs are tricky for me to remove, but this can has always been easy for me to open. I used a spoon to scoop the meat and gravy over the dry cat food. It smelled almost like a Sunday dinner.

Toby was getting hungry. I could tell because he was walking back and forth in front of his food area. I placed the bowl in its spot. Toby looked at me and meowed again.

"You are very welcome, Toby," I said.

I watched Toby for a minute to make sure he was not eating too fast. I remembered that cats could get sick if they eat too fast. Today he was taking his time and enjoying his breakfast. He licked his mouth and chewed each bite.

While he was eating, I finished cleaning up our breakfast mess. The can went into the waste bin. I took a washcloth and wiped the crumbs off the counter.

Even though I took care of Toby's breakfast, I still felt like there was more that I had to do today. I looked at Toby again to see if there was anything that he could remind me to do. He did not give me any new ideas.

I looked at the cabinets again. He had plenty of food for the next few days, so I didn't need to go to the store for him.

I went to the calendar that was posted by the refrigerator. It had a colorful photo of a large tree with bright fall colors. The boxes under the photo had writing for each day.

All the days that were done had an X crossed through them. Today's date had an appointment written on it.

"Oh look, Toby," I said to my cat. "It looks like you are visiting the doctor today."

Toby just meowed and walked out of the kitchen.

chapter 3
Playing With Toby

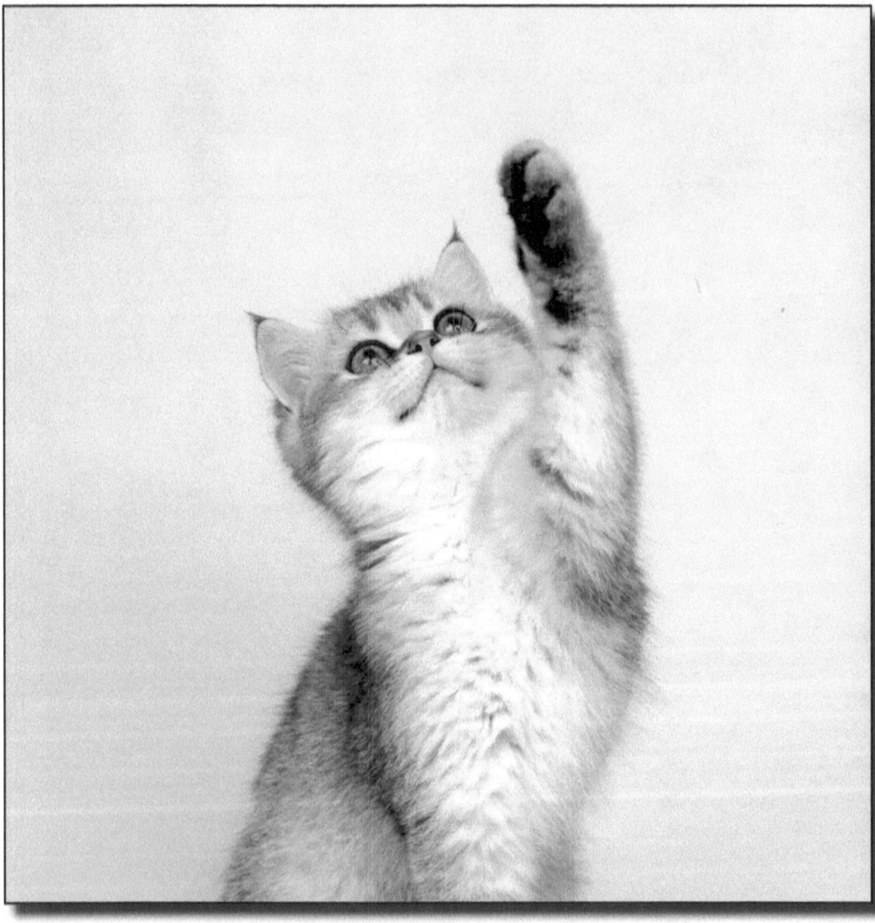

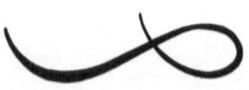

TOBY'S APPOINTMENT with the vet was not for another few hours. Now that we both had something to eat, it was time for us to do something while we waited.

I gave Toby a chance to finish his breakfast without me watching the whole time. I went back to my bedroom to change into my clothes for the day. I found a pair of blue slacks, a gray t-shirt, and a sweater jacket. I already had my socks on, so my feet were warm enough.

After I was dressed, I put on my slip-on shoes and went outside to my mailbox. The mail was not there, but the newspaper was in its slot under the mailbox. I knew many people who are reading the news on their computers and phones. I can find what I am looking for in the real paper.

I took my newspaper to the living room and settled in my chair. Toby meowed to let me know that he was in the room with me. He walked over to the tower by the bookshelf and started scratching the carpet on it.

It had been a while since Toby climbed the cat tower. I don't remember the last time he climbed to the top when the sun was shining on it. Maybe that is something I should ask the doctor about today.

I read through the first section of the newspaper. It was the latest news from the country and the world. It also had stories of people and places in my town. There were plenty of ads and stories about the upcoming election too.

I was near the end of the newspaper section when something tapped the bottom edge of the paper. I put the newspaper down to see Toby next to me. He used the ramp on the cat tower to climb to the window seat, then jump over to the side table.

"Does Toby need attention?" I asked my cat friend. He walked on top of the newspaper on my lap and sat on top of it.

I could not resist scratching Toby behind his ears. He started to purr and rub his head against my fingers. He wanted to make sure that I scratched the right spot.

"Yes," I told Toby, "just a little attention." The vibrations from his purring made the paper under him rattle and crinkle. I was almost done with that section, so I did not mind.

Toby used his paw to touch the hand I was scratching his head with. That was his sign to stop. I put that hand back on the armrest. After a few moments, I reached over to the basket of Toby's toys. I kept it next to my chair so that I could reach it at times like these.

My hand grabbed one of his favorite toys. Once I had a good grip, I started to click the button. A red light appeared on the floor.

Toby knew what the clicking sound meant. He stood up on my lap and carefully walked down my legs. Once he found the red light, he jumped on it, trying to catch it.

I turned off the red light from the laser pointer and watched Toby look around for the light. I clicked it back on and pointed to another part of the floor. Toby jumped up and tried to catch it again.

Toby was having fun chasing this moving target and I was having fun giving him something to do. I liked to change where the light would show up next and see if he could find it.

After a while, Toby was getting bored with our game. When I started to shine the light somewhere else, he walked over to his cat tower and started cleaning himself. I put the red light away in the basket while he licked the fur on his back leg.

I went back to my newspaper to finish reading. Toby decided to take a little cat nap after all of his playing.

I got up from my chair to wash a load of laundry. Toby was too comfortable to follow me. It did not take me long before I was back in my chair with a fresh cup of coffee.

I checked my watch. There was still about 2 hours before Toby's appointment. I knew I was not driving us there. I was just beginning to wonder when Mia was going to show up.

At that point, I heard a knock on the front door. Toby's head popped up to see what was going on, but the rest of his body stayed in its cozy spot on the floor.

"Don't worry, Toby," I told my cat. "I think it is just your friend at the door."

chapter 4
Time For A Road Trip

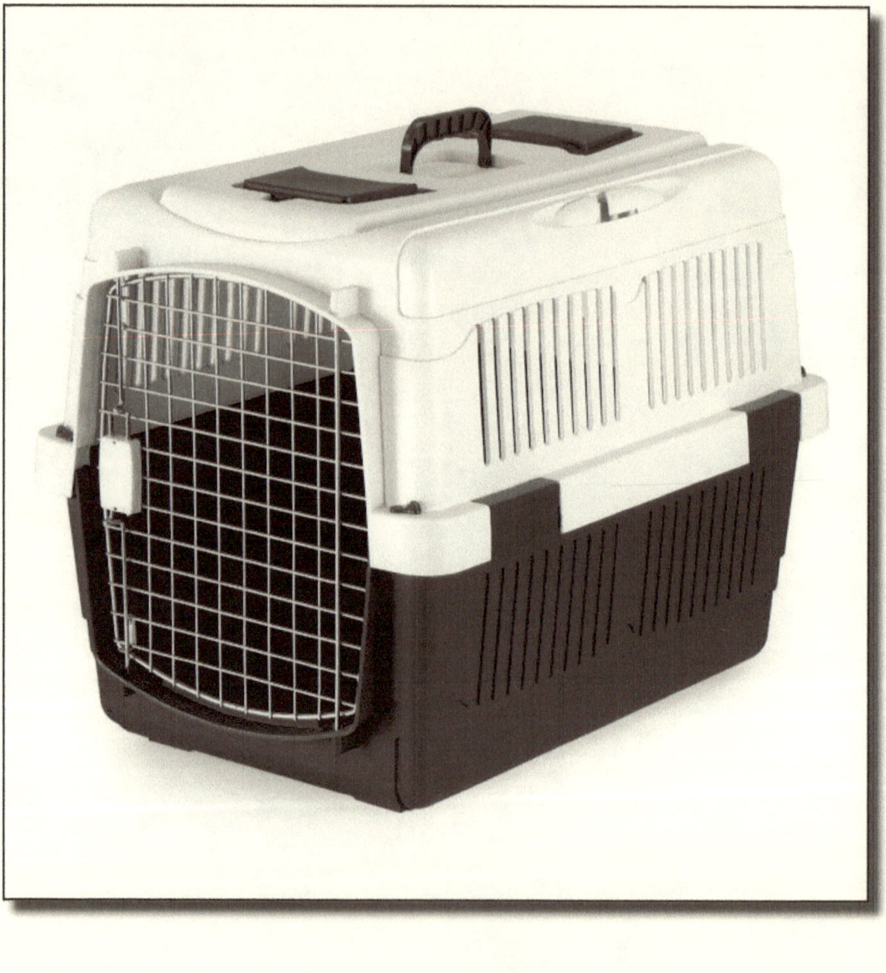

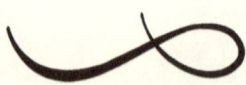

I WALKED to the front door and opened it for our visitor.

"Hi, Ma," my daughter Mia greeted me. Mia had two cloth bags in her hands. She gave me a quick hug before she walked through the doorway.

"Hi, Mia." We walked toward the kitchen where she set the bags down on the counter.

"I found some cat food on sale so I got a few extra cans for Toby," Mia said. She started removing cans from her bags and putting them on the shelves with the rest of the cat food.

"Sounds good," I said. "Toby will be happy with that.

At that moment, Toby walked into the kitchen and started to rub against Mia's legs.

"Well, good morning to you too, sir," Mia said with a smile. She was the one who helped me adopt Toby so that I could have a friend in my house. I always thought that Toby was just as much her pet as he was mine.

"We have Toby's vet appointment at 11:00," I reminded Mia as I handed her some of the cat treats that were in the bag I helped empty.

"Yup," she replied. "We are still on schedule." She folded her bag before she got to her knees to pet Toby behind the ears.

Toby loved all the extra attention he got from Mia. I think he knew that she was the one who got him the special treats and toys.

Mia looked up at me. "Are you ready to go?" she asked.

"Yes," I answered. "I have a list of what he eats in case they ask.

"Then I better get this fellow ready, too," Mia said. When Mia stood up, Toby moved over to his food dish and had a snack.

Mia went to the laundry room and brought out Toby's carrier. The vet's office can be very busy with other animals who have appointments and emergency visits. Since Toby and other cats do not use a leash like dogs can, it is easier to keep him calm and safe in a travel carrier.

She set the carrier on the floor and placed a furry toy mouse in the carrier. She also added a catnip toy so that he had something to keep him busy and comfortable.

"Toby, it is time for a road trip," Mia called out to my cat.

Toby looked up from his food bowl and yawned a huge yawn. He then placed his front paws forward, put his tail straight into the air, and stretched a huge stretch.

He took his time walking over to the carrier. He looked inside, saw his favorite toys, and walked in. When Mia closed the door to the carrier, I could see that he was pawing the cushion on the bottom of the carrier. He was getting ready to go.

Mia picked up the carrier. I'm glad she did. Even though Toby can be lightweight, the carrier is so big that it can be awkward for me to carry. I grabbed my bag with Toby's items and followed Mia out the door.

"Do I have the key?" I asked myself out loud. I had my keys in my hand and locked the door behind me. "Yes, I have my key."

For years, I always asked myself questions like this. The one time that I didn't, I had locked myself out of the house until Mia was able to bring her key and let me in.

Mia was putting Toby and his carrier in the back of her car. I put my keys in my bag and went to her car. The door on the passenger side was unlocked so I sat down and buckled my seatbelt.

Mia did the same in the driver's seat and started the car. "See?" she said to me. "We are still on schedule."

"I remember the first time we tried to get Toby in the carrier," I told Mia as she started driving. "He did not want to be cooped up in that box until he had all of the snacks and toys that he could ever want."

"It took us at least 15 minutes before he finally agreed," Mia replied. "I'm glad he is a little more mellow about the carrier now."

"Me, too," I said. Toby used to have more energy when he was younger. He was a handful back then, but we got so used to each other that I am happy for these easier times.

Toby's vet was not far from my house, so it did not take long to get to the vet's office. We pulled into the parking lot 20 minutes before our scheduled appointment.

"Alright, Toby," Mia called to the back of her car. "Dr. Sharp will be ready to see you.

All I could hear was one little "meow" come out of the carrier.

chapter 5
Dr. Sharp

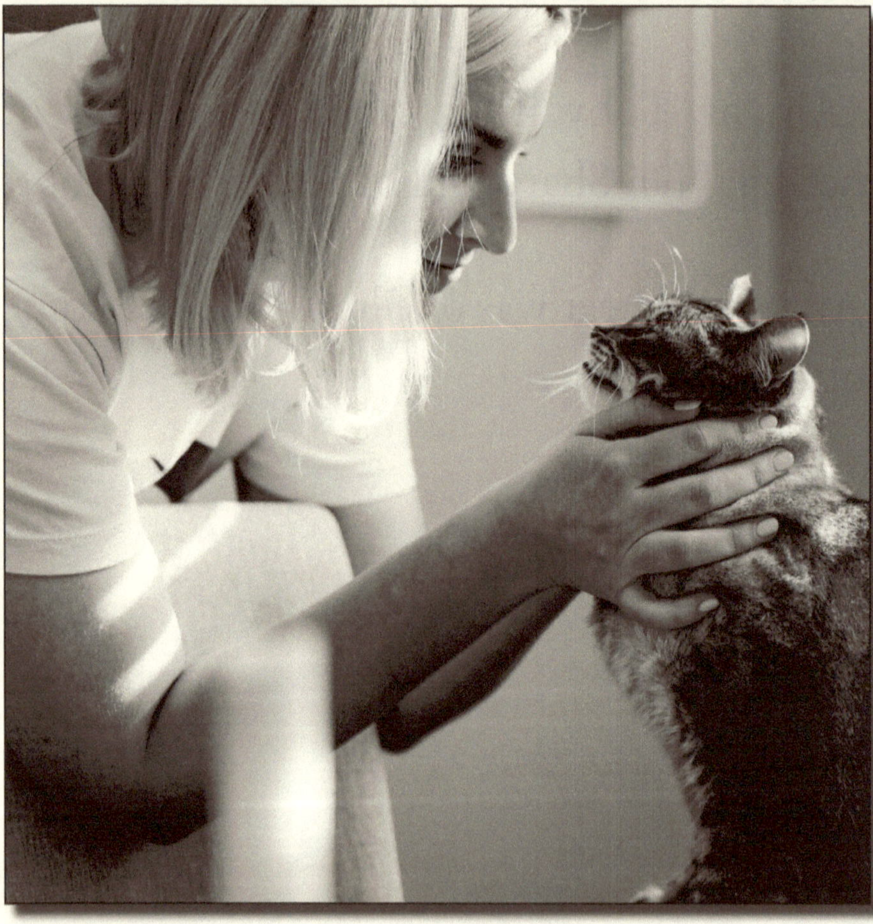

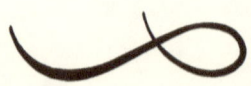

THE WAITING ROOM for the vet was noisy with all sorts of pets. Dogs and cats were in carriers like Toby. Some were on a leash sitting next to their owner.

As we walked in, there were barks that greeted us. Some barks were loud and deep, and some were high and constant. Every now and then I heard something that sounded like a bird, but I could not see where it was.

We got in line to see the lady at the counter. "How can I help you today?"

Mia spoke up. "Toby has an appointment with Dr. Sharp."

"Great," the lady said. She handed Mia a clipboard with some papers under her window. "If you can update Toby's information and any concerns you have today, we will get you to the back as soon as we can."

There were two seats by the window. We sat down and I started to fill out the information on the paper. There were questions about food, vitamins, and if Toby was acting differently.

Some of the answers were already filled out, like birthday and address. It was easy to check off those facts and not write everything.

When I was finished with the papers, I gave the clipboard back to the lady behind the window. She smiled and put them in a stack with other clipboards. I sat down and waited for our turn.

The waiting room was a big space. It helped keep all the animals in their own space. I could see that some of the dogs on leashes were friendly with each other. Their owners seemed to know each other since they were talking to each other.

Other animals were kept quiet by staying in their carriers or on their owner's laps. I looked into Toby's carrier to see how he was doing. All I saw was the back of his head and I assumed he was taking another cat nap.

Some of the animals were called to the back room. I liked some of their names like "Steak" for a big, strong dog or Cupcake for a black cat with white fur on top. Finally, I heard "Toby" called out.

We followed the lady to one of the back rooms. It was a small vet office, but everyone was always helpful and friendly with the animals.

"How are you today?" she smiled. "Bring the carrier to the table and we will see if Toby is ready to come out."

Mia placed the carrier on the metal table then opened the carrier door. Toby took one step forward and stretched out to make his body as long as he could. He had a lot of space in his carrier, but I was sure it felt good to be able to move everywhere again.

Dr. Sharp came into the exam room. She was looking at some papers on a clipboard.

"Good morning, everyone," the doctor looked up at us and smiled. "How are we doing?

Dr. Sharp put the paperwork down and started to examine Toby. She stroked his fur and felt his muscles and bones. "So, our big boy is 9 years old, correct?" she asked.

"Yes," I answered. I remembered that number from the paperwork.

Dr. Sharp took a pen light and looked in Toby's eyes and ears. "That means that he is considered a senior cat now. Have you ever had a senior cat before?" she asked.

"Sure," I told the doctor. "They get slower and need a little more attention. Like right now I know that Toby does not like to climb his tower anymore. He also seems to sleep more, but still plays with some of his toys."

"That's right," Dr. Sharp said. "Changes in weight are also important to look for." The doctor looked at the vet tech who was weighing Toby on the scale in the room. "How much is Toby today?"

"Ten pounds," the nurse said. She brought Toby back to the table.

"Still a good weight," the doctor said. "His diet is working well, so keep with what you are doing." She listened to Toby's heart and lungs next. Toby purred against the doctor. I was not sure how she could hear his heart with all of that noise.

"Toby looks good. At this point, schedule another appointment for six months and we will also get some lab work done at that time as well. Any questions?" the doctor asked me.

I looked at Mia who was helping Toby back into the carrier. "I don't think so," I said.

"Just be sure to call if you notice any changes. We can help more if we find problems sooner." Dr. Sharp said. She shook my hand and went to the next room for her next appointment.

The vet tech walked us out to the counter so that we could make the next appointment for six months. After that, it was time to go home.

chapter 6
Back At Home

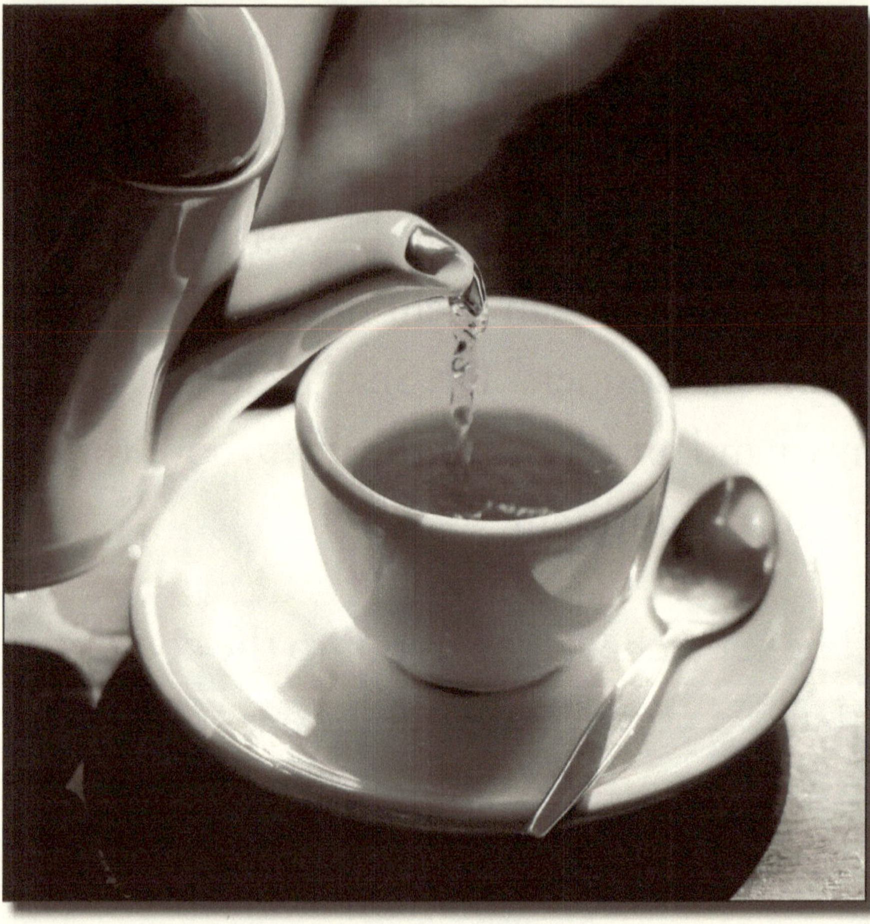

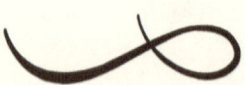

WHEN WE arrived home, I unlocked the door for Mia. She brought the carrier with Toby into the house.

She set the carrier down and opened the gate. Toby did not come out right away, so we left him to come out when he was ready.

"Do you want some tea, Ma?" Mia asked.

"Sure, I'll get the mugs," I offered.

Mia filled the kettle with water and put it on the stovetop. I picked two blue mugs from the cabinet. Next, I picked the box of tea bags from the pantry.

When the kettle started to whistle, I heard Toby meow to the loud sound.

"I know you don't like tea or loud noise, Toby," I told my cat. "How about a little treat instead?"

I took a cat treat from the pantry as well as the tea. He enjoyed that snack even more after Mia took the kettle off the heat.

"So, Toby is a senior, just like me," I said to Mia. We sat down at the table to drink our tea.

"Yes," Mia said. She tried to sip her tea, but it was still too hot for her. "A wise old man with a few of his nine lives left."

"Oh please," I said. "Toby has been such a good boy. I am sure that he has many of those lives."

I looked over at Toby who was rolling around on the floor. He was playing with the mouse toy that I stepped on this morning.

"I am just happy that he is healthy, and we don't have to change anything yet," I said to Mia.

Mia nodded. "You feed him right, and his toys are right for his age. The ramp even helps him get up and down instead of jumping. We don't want him to get hurt."

"I know I want a few more years with Toby," I said.

Toby meowed when he heard his name.

"I think he is on the right track for that," Mia said as she sipped her tea.

"Speaking of eating right, I think it is time for his dinner," I said.

I stood up and did the same thing that I did for his breakfast. First, I cleaned the bowls. Then I refilled the water. Finally, I scooped the right amount of food to keep him happy.

Mia stood up and put her mug in the sink. "It looks like you have everything set. I need to get back home to see my kids."

"Send them my love," I hugged Mia. "Thank you for taking Toby and me to the vet today."

"Anytime, Ma." She grabbed her bags and left.

The house was quiet again, so I turned on the radio to play some music for Toby and me. I washed the tea mugs and put them back on the shelf.

"I think it is time for me to have something to eat as well," I told Toby. He was too busy chewing on his food.

I put some chicken soup in a small pot and turned on the stove. I made the soup a few days ago so all I had to do was warm it up. When it was ready, I poured it in a soup mug and took it to the table again.

"It looks like we finished everything we had to do today. What do you think, Toby?" I asked my friend.

Toby walked over to where I was sitting and rubbed against my leg. I loved his little hugs like that.

"Ok, maybe not everything," I said.

After I cleaned up my meal, I turned off the music and the light in the kitchen. We went back to my favorite chair. I carefully picked up Toby and placed him on my lap.

"Just a quick brush today," I told Toby. Every week I made sure to brush Toby's fur. He did a good job cleaning himself. I just make sure that I get some of the extra fur.

I took the brush out of the basket and started to gently comb his fur. I started from between his ears and brushed down his back. I stopped at his tail and brushed again.

Toby did not have long fur, so it was easy for me to keep him brushed.

Toby purred and purred. He liked being brushed so it was one of his favorite times of the day. It was a time that I enjoy with Toby as well.

When I was done brushing Toby, I put the brush away and scratched him under his chin. He was a good companion.

"Well, Toby," I said out loud. "I don't know if we have to do anything tomorrow. Is there anything you want to do?"

Toby meowed and put his head down on his paws.

"I agree," I told him. "No doctors. We should just do whatever we want."

And we did.   THE END

The Cat Appointment – Chapter Summaries

Chapter 1 – Something To Do

From the moment I woke up, I felt a sense of purpose. I slowly walk around my home, noticing small details. As I drink my coffee I greet my cat...

Chapter 2 – Feeding Toby

While enjoying my cereal and milk, I watch my cat playing on the kitchen floor. This triggers memories of the various cats in my life. After I have prepared Toby's food, I look at my calendar and realize it is his vet appointment today...

Chapter 3 – Playing With Toby

I get dressed and bring in the newspaper from the mailbox. I entertain Toby with a laser pointer and watch him chase the red light. Toby takes a nap while I do my household chores...

Chapter 4 – Time For A Road Trip

My daughter, Mia, arrives bringing cans of pet food with her. We make sure Toby is safe in his travel carrier for the journey by car to the vet's office...

Chapter 5 – Dr. Sharp

The vet's waiting room is busy with all kinds of pets. I complete paperwork before we see Dr. Sharp. She carefully examines Toby who confirms he is in good health...

Chapter 6 – Back At Home

We make tea after arriving back home. I talk about how Toby is a wise old cat. After Mia leaves, I listen to the radio and reheat chicken soup for my evening meal. After cleaning up I gently brush Toby's fur and listen to him purr...

THE END

SHORT STORIES

Delightful short stories
all about cats

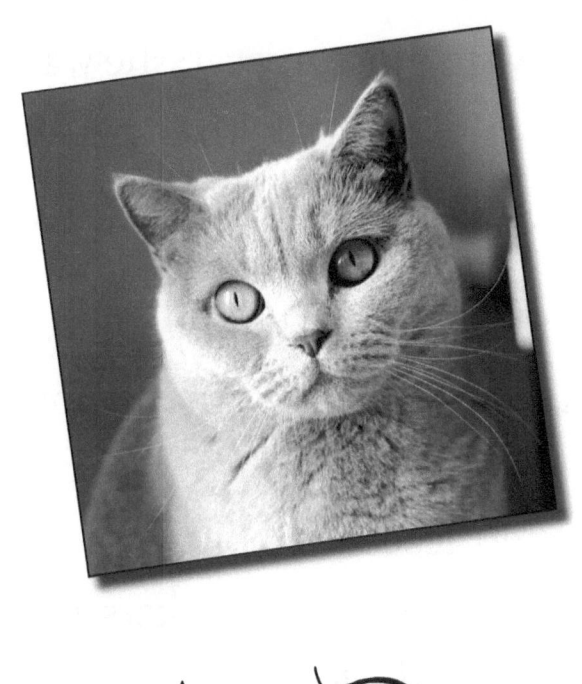

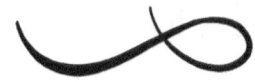

Short Story 1
The Senior Center Cat

AT THE Rosewood Senior Center there was a weekly event that everyone looked forward to with eager anticipation. It was the day the therapy cat, Whiskers, came to visit.

Whiskers wasn't just any cat; she was a fluffy, gray-and-white feline with a personality as warm as a summer's day.

Every Thursday, the seniors at Rosewood gathered in the cozy common room, where comfortable chairs formed a circle around the centerpiece—a plush, cushioned armchair reserved for Whiskers the cat. As the clock ticked closer to her arrival, the room buzzed with excitement.

Mrs. Jenkins was usually the first to spot the familiar sight of Whiskers' carrier being wheeled in by the volunteer, Sarah. The mere glimpse of the carrier set off a chain reaction of smiles and chuckles among the residents. Sarah, with a twinkle in her eye, would slowly open the carrier door, and out would strut Whiskers, her tail held high, and her eyes full of affection.

Whiskers had the ability to sense who needed her attention the most. For example, she'd make her way to Mr. Anderson, who often struggled with loneliness. Curling up on his lap, she'd nuzzle against his wrinkled hands. It was as if Whiskers could sense the need to lift him out of solitude.

Mrs. Thompson was a bubbly woman who had danced her way through life. She'd sing old tunes, and Whiskers would purr in perfect harmony. Their duets brought smiles to those who listened and encouraged them to join in.

As Whiskers moved from person to person, she left a trail of positivity in her wake. The once-quiet room became filled with laughter and storytelling of fondly remembered pets. Residents began to open up and live in the moment.

Whiskers was not just a therapy cat, she was a catalyst for happiness and companionship. She forged bonds among the seniors, reminding them of the beauty in simple moments and the joy of shared connections. Her presence was a weekly reminder that love, in its purest form, could come in the soft, furry package of a cat.

Whiskers had taught them that no matter how old you grew, there was always room for happiness and positivity. Sometimes all it took was a little feline friend to make that lesson clear.   THE END

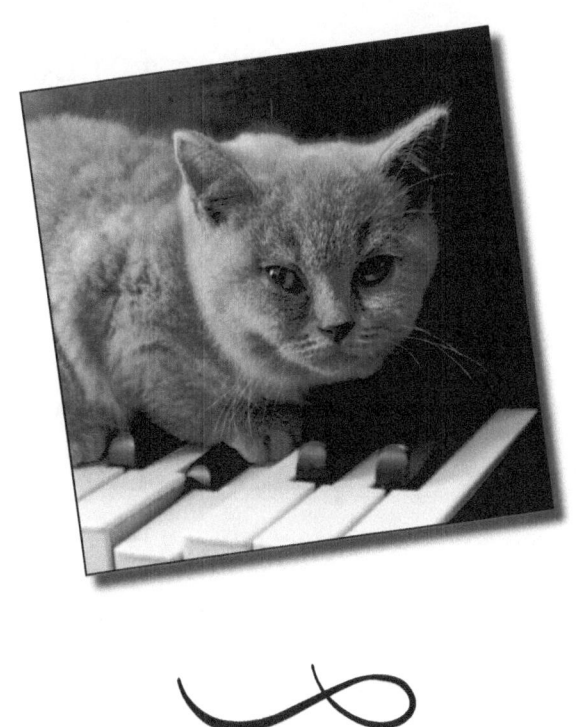

Short Story 2
The Jazz Emporium's Cat

IN THE heart of New Orleans, a retired jazz musician named Max had a dream: to create a haven where the spirit of jazz would live on in the form of antique musical instruments.

"The Jazz Emporium" was a unique shop echoed with the sweet melodies of the past. It also had an enchanting cat ambassador, named Louis.

Max had once traveled the world as a working jazz saxophonist, but with the passing of time, he decided to return to his beloved hometown and pursue his other passion – collecting antique musical instruments. Louis, a relaxed smokey cat with wise eyes, became his loyal companion.

The shop was a treasure trove of instruments – saxophones, trumpets, clarinets, pianos, harmonicas and more Each piece reflecting the soul of jazz. But what truly set "The Jazz Emporium" apart was Louis. He was a natural entertainer and a jazz aficionado in his own way.

Tourists and locals alike flocked to the shop, not just for the exquisite instruments but also for the soothing presence of Louis. As you entered, you were serenaded by the sounds of Max's saxophone, and there was Loius, poised on a velvet cushion, his eyes shimmering with a hint of mischief.

Louis seemed to be able to sense the rhythm of the music. He'd often choose a particular instrument to 'play' alongside Max, swatting gently at the keys or strings, adding his own delightful feline touch to the performance.

Max's shop gained a reputation, and other musicians would come and jam along with them. It wasn't long before a documentary crew arrived to capture the unique partnership between Max and Louis. The resulting film was seen around the world and was given international awards. Soon, "The Jazz Emporium" became a must-visit destination for jazz enthusiasts and curious travelers.

Max and Louis remained true to their roots. The true essence of jazz was about spontaneous improvisation, collaboration, and the joy it brought to people's lives.

"The Jazz Emporium" was a testament to the enduring magic of music and the deep bond between an aging jazz musician and his extraordinary cat friend. Together, they kept the soul of jazz alive, one note at a time.

THE END

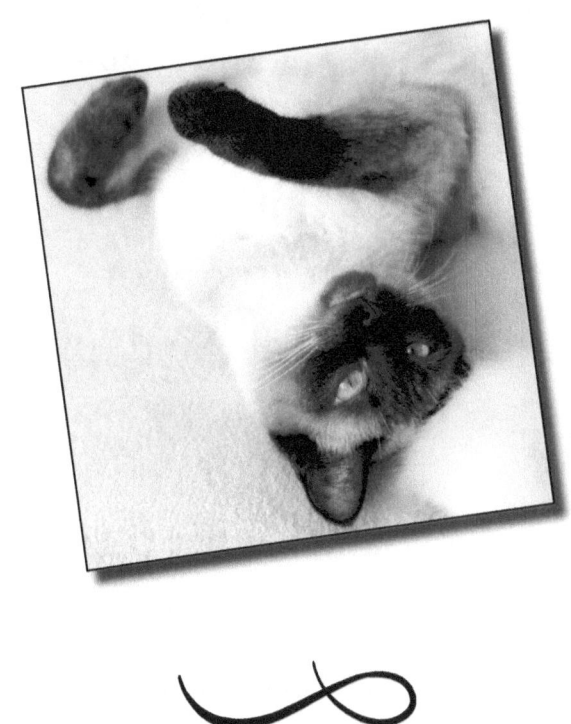

Short Story 3
The Dance Partner

IN THE bustling heart of New York City, on the upper floor of a charming apartment building, lived an elderly woman named Heidi. She had spent her youth as a passionate dancer, gracing stages with her grace and beauty. Now, in her golden years, she had traded the dance floor for a quiet apartment and danced no more. That was until she met her agile and playful cat, Apollo.

Apollo, a sleek and elegant Siamese cat, arrived in Heidi's life as a kitten. He brought with him an exuberance for life that was infectious. As Heidi watched him prance around their cozy living room, she felt a familiar spark reignite within her. It was the call of the dance.

Heidi's love for dance had never truly faded from her heart. It had just taken a back seat to the demands of life and the aging process. Now, with Apollo as her dance partner, she was ready to relive her passion. She put on some of her favorite music, and the two began to gently move and twirl around the living room, creating their own dance routine.

Their dance sessions became a regular event, with Eleanor and Apollo swaying to the rhythms of various genres, from classical waltzes to lively jazz tunes. Apollo, with his nimble movements, leaped and twirled in perfect harmony with his owner. The living room was transformed into their private stage, where life's worries disappeared, and they celebrated the joy of movement.

As their dance sessions continued, Heidi discovered new ways that her aging body express itself. The fluid motions or her youth were now replaced by slower movements that still graceful and followed gentler rhythms. It was all thanks to her dedicated partner, Apollo. Their dances showed the enduring beauty of dance and the power of companionship.

One evening, as they moved to the mesmerizing melodies of a tango, Heidi's neighbor from the floor below paid them a visit. She wanted to meet the remarkable dancer whose movements she could hear.

Heidi's neighbor turned out to be a piano teacher and offered to play the piano while Heidi and Apollo danced. The neighbor was able to adapt the tempo and style of famous music to better suite their dances.

Heidi and Apollo continued to dance their way through life, a welcome reminder that it's never too late to rekindle one's love for the arts and to celebrate life through dance, music and movement.

THE END

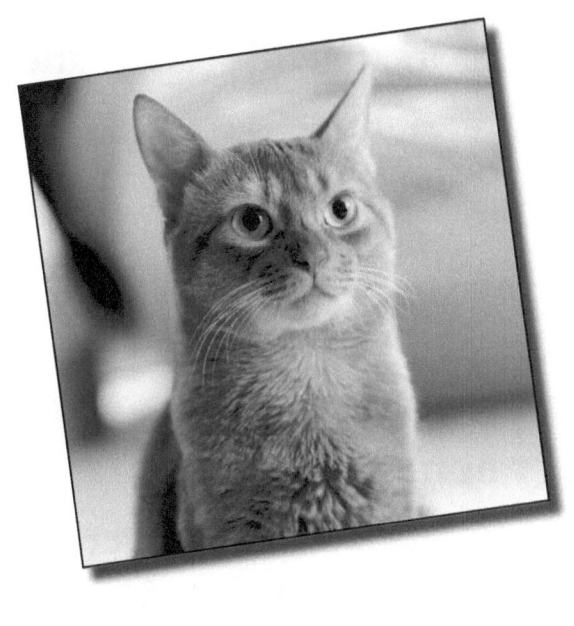

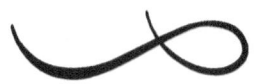

Short Story 4
The Cat and the
Reading Club

IN A QUIET suburban neighborhood, a retiree named Margaret decided to embark on a new venture in her golden years. She had always been an avid reader, and felt the time was now right to start a neighborhood book club. What made her club truly unique, however, was the presence of her beloved cat, Mr. Felix.

Margaret's home was a warm and inviting place where fellow book lovers gathered, their cozy circle of armchairs and sofas surrounding a coffee table stacked high with novels. Mr. Felix, a charming orange tabby with bright green eyes, was a friendly presence, curling up in a corner or playfully chasing a sunbeam.

At the first book club meeting, Margaret introduced Mr. Felix to the group. The members were initially surprised but soon charmed by the cat's endearing antics and calm demeanor. Mr. Felix had an ability to look as if he was really listening to whoever was sharing their thoughts about a book. He would look attentive and often perch on their laps.

As the months went by, Margaret's book club flourished, and it was not just because of the engaging discussions. Mr. Felix had become a beloved member in his own right. His presence added a unique charm and sense of camaraderie to the club, and his quiet purring seemed to encourage deeper conversations and added to the relaxed atmosphere.

The club meetings often stretched into warm afternoons, with members discussing books, life, and sharing personal stories, all while enjoying the company of their furry friend. Mr. Felix' playful antics, like chasing imaginary mice or performing acrobatic leaps, would elicit laughter and serve as a delightful icebreaker.

Outside of book club meetings, Margaret and Mr. Felix were often seen taking leisurely strolls, visiting local cafes, or simply enjoying the sunshine in their backyard. Neighbors and passersby would smile at the sight of Margaret and Mr. Felix together.

The book club meetings showed that the love of books and the warmth of friendships were ageless and timeless, and that sometimes, all it took was a little cat to bring people together.

THE END

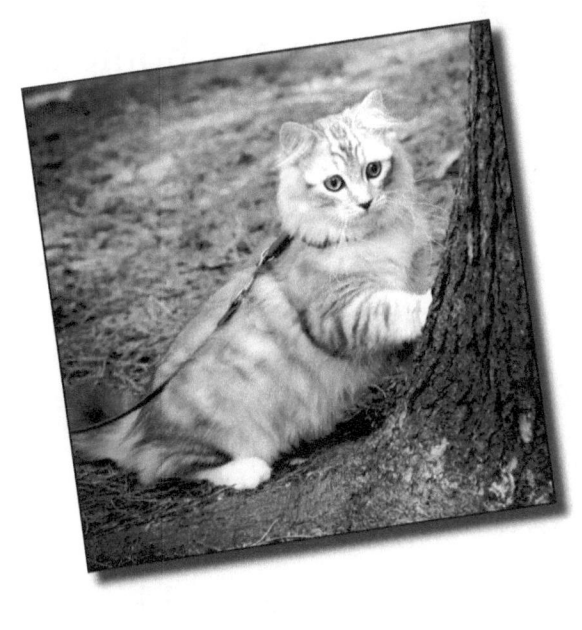

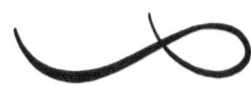

Short Story 5
Maine Cat Adventures

IN THE picturesque coastal town of Bar Harbor, Maine, Robert, a retiree, found himself entering a new phase of life. He had always dreamed of taking the time to really explore the beauty of his home state, and now, with the companionship of his adventurous cat, Luna, he was ready to embark on a series of memorable adventures.

Their first journey took them to the rocky shores of Acadia National Park. Luna, with her playful spirit, scampered along the craggy cliffs, but Robert had her on a leash, ensuring she stayed close. As she chased seagulls that soared overhead, Robert couldn't help but smile as he watched his feline friend delight in the fresh sea air while keeping her safe.

Their next destination was Bass Harbor Head Lighthouse, a symbol of Maine's maritime history. Luna perched on a nearby rock, her eyes filled with curiosity as they watched the waves crash against the rugged coastline. Robert imagined the countless ships that had been guided safely by the lighthouse's guiding beacon over the years, all while Luna explored the area under his watchful gaze.

With each adventure, Luna's playful antics and zest for life breathed new energy into Robert. They ventured into charming coastal villages like Camden and Rockland, where they explored quaint shops, enjoyed seafood delicacies, and discovered the rich maritime heritage of Maine. Luna's leash allowed her to accompany Robert on his explorations, keeping her close and ensuring her safety while they reveled in the coastal charm.

Their travels continued inland to the tranquil lakes of Maine, where they spent quiet afternoons by the water's edge, watching the reflection of the surrounding forests on the serene surface. Luna, with her tail lazily swaying, would keep a watchful eye on the birds that played in the trees above, enjoying the beauty of the outdoors while staying close to her beloved companion.

The pair ventured into the woods of Baxter State Park, where the scent of pine and the sound of rustling leaves were a soothing balm to their souls. Robert imagined the years melt away as he gently hiked through the pristine wilderness, and Luna, with her keen instincts, would occasionally lead the way with boundless energy.

In the town of Rangeley, they explored Saddleback Lake, one of Maine's hidden gems. Luna explored the water's edge with enthusiasm, her natural grace mirrored in the ripples she created. Robert watched, savoring the beauty of the moment.

Their travels took them to the summit of Mount Katahdin, the tallest peak in Maine. As they stood at the base, Robert took a photographed and marveled at natural beauty of the landscape. Luna sat beside him, her tail brushing against his leg, as if to share in the quiet contemplation.

In their travels throughout Maine, they celebrated the beauty of their home state. Robert and Luna's journeys showed that it's never too late to embrace the wonders of life when you have an adventurous spirit by your side.

THE END

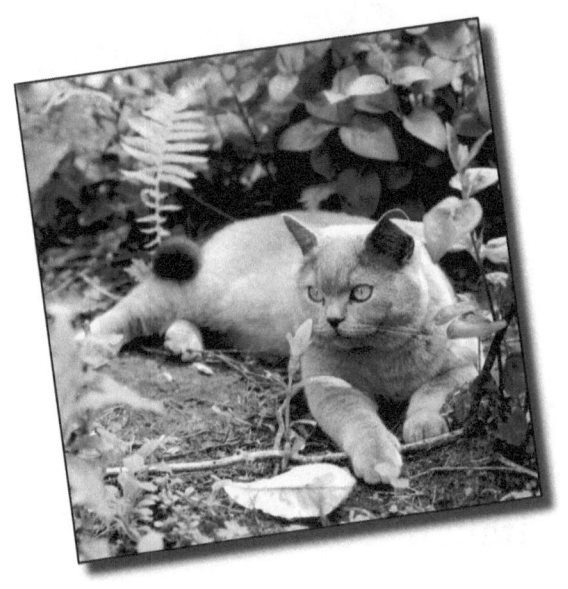

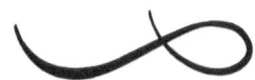

Short Story 6
The Garden Companion

IN THE countryside of Tuscany, Italy, a tranquil villa was home to an elderly woman named Rosa. She had always cherished the idea of spending her retirement days amidst the rolling vineyards and fragrant gardens of Italy. Her dream came true when she moved to this picturesque landscape and began tending to a beautiful garden, with her faithful cat, Bianca, by her side.

Rosa had a love for nature and gardening, and the Italian countryside provided the perfect backdrop for her passion. Her garden was a special place where she could immerse herself in the vibrant colors and fragrant blooms that surrounded her. As she pruned, planted, and weeded, Bianca was her ever-present companion, watching with curiosity and occasionally chasing after butterflies that danced in the warm Italian sun.

Their days began with the soft, golden light of the Italian sunrise. Rosa would step into her garden, and Bianca would follow, her dainty paws brushing against the dew-kissed grass. Together, they inspected the garden's progress, checking for new buds, admiring blossoms, and ensuring that each plant thrived under their care.

Bianca would find the sunniest spot in the garden, where she would stretch out and bask in the warmth, occasionally casting a watchful eye over Rosa as she worked. Her presence was a soothing constant, a reminder that Rosa was never truly alone in this beautiful corner of Italy.

As the seasons changed, the garden transformed into a kaleidoscope of colors and scents. Roses, lavender, and sunflowers painted a vivid picture, attracting the gentle buzz of bees and the fluttering of butterflies.

The garden also attracted local birds, and Rosa and Bianca spent hours watching them flit among the olive trees, the birdsong filling the air.

In the afternoons, Rosa would sit on a rustic bench, sipping espresso while Bianca nestled in her lap. They would watch the world go by, enjoying the simple beauty of life and the bond they had forged amidst the Tuscan countryside.

Bianca's playful antics added joy to Rosa's gardening routine. She would occasionally pounce on fallen leaves or chase after a playful butterfly, her agility and grace entertaining her owner. Her laughter echoed through the garden, a reminder that age was no barrier to finding joy in life's simple pleasures.

As evening descended upon the Italian countryside, Rosa and Bianca would retreat to their villa, tired but content. Rosa would stroke Bianca's soft fur, feeling the comforting rhythm of her purring. The garden outside whispered with the secrets of nature, and the two companions would drift into slumber, dreaming of another day filled with the beauty of their Italian haven.

Their garden flourished with vibrant colors and life, reflecting the love, care, and joy they shared, and reminding them that life's true treasures could often be found in the simplest of moments.

THE END

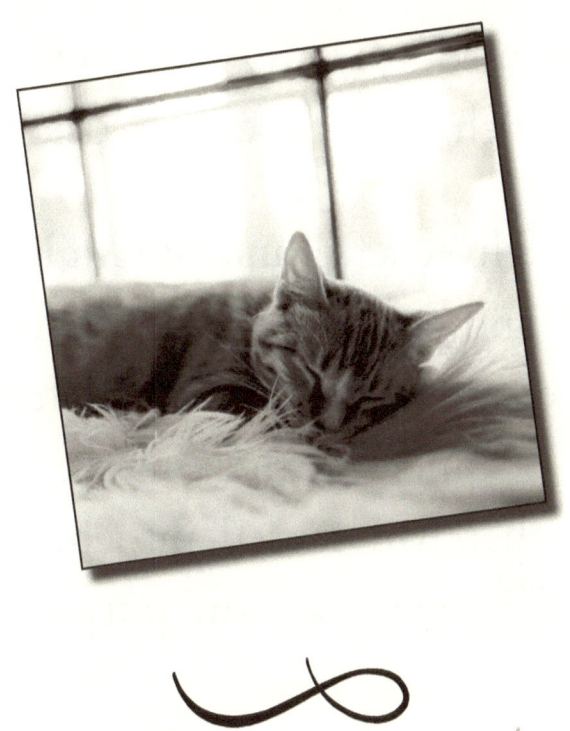

Short Story 7
The Cat Café

IN THE HEART of the city, amidst the hustle and bustle of everyday life, there was a charming cat cafe. It was here that an elderly man named Henry found solace, companionship, and a sense of belonging.

Henry had lived a full and vibrant life, but as he aged and his family moved away, he found he was a little lonely. Each day had become a quiet routine, marked by the solitude that had settled into his life. He yearned for connection and purpose.

One afternoon, while taking a leisurely stroll through the city, Henry happened upon the Cat Cafe. Its large windows allowed him to peer inside, where he saw a group of cats of all shapes and sizes, playfully chasing toys and curling up in cozy nooks. The sight was so unexpected that he had to enter and find out more.

Inside, he was greeted by the inviting aroma of fresh coffee and the soothing purrs of the resident cat companions. He heard soft laughter and conversation as patrons, young and old, sipped their drinks and interacted with the cats. It was wonderful.

Henry, a lover of cats from his younger years, found himself drawn to a calico named Marmalade. He reached out to stroke her, and she responded with a gentle head nuzzle. It was a simple moment that filled Henry's heart with a sense of connection he had sorely missed.

It reminded him of when he was a young boy. As a child, he had spent countless hours playing with their farm cat by the warm fireplace. It was a friendly kitten, similar to Marmalade, that always seemed to be darting about, chasing after shadows, and pouncing on imaginary prey. The warmth of the crackling fire and the purring of the farm cat were happy memories of his childhood.

From that day forward, Henry became a regular at the Cat Cafe. He would visit every day, sitting by the window with Marmalade in his lap, as if they were old friends. The cafe's patrons soon became familiar with him, and he struck up conversations with others who shared a love for cats. He found a sense of belonging within the cozy cafe walls.

The Cat Cafe gave him not only the company of Marmalade but also the company of kindred spirits. He felt that he was part of a community. It became a source of daily joy, and a reminder that loneliness could be replaced with shared moments of warmth and connection.

Henry had discovered that sometimes, companionship and comfort could be found in the most unexpected places, and that a simple cup of coffee and a playful cat could bring light and laughter back into his life.

THE END

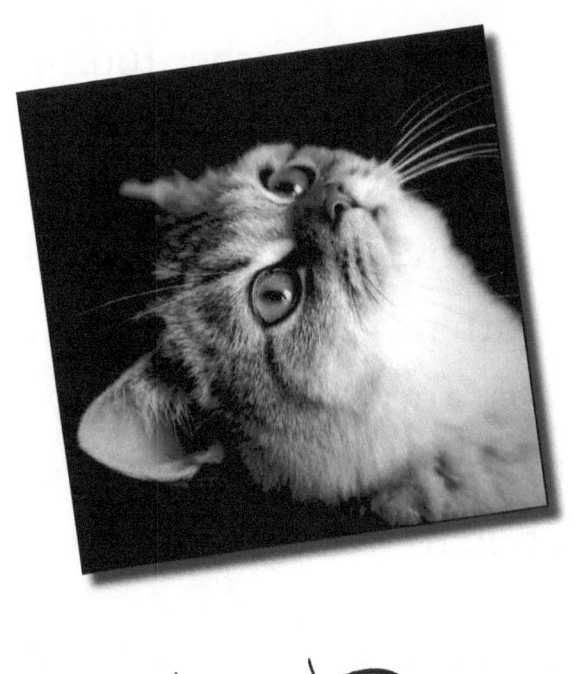

Short Story 8
Choosing Lucky

HANNAH, a bright-eyed little girl, skipped along the cobblestone street towards the local pet shop. It was a sunny Saturday morning. Her grandmother Judith held her hand, sharing in Hannah's excitement.

The pet shop was a wonderland filled with adorable kittens, playful puppies, and all manner of furry and feathery friends. Today, their mission was clear: to find the perfect kitten to welcome into their home.

Judith had always loved animals and decided that it was time to add a new member to their family. She wanted Hannah to experience the joy of caring for a pet, just as she had with her own grandmother many years ago.

There was a cheerful bell jingle from the door as they entered the shop. Row after row of furry faces peered out from behind glass enclosures. Hannah's eyes widened, and her heart swelled with anticipation.

The pair began to explore the different kittens in search of their new family member. Hannah was drawn to a playful tabby with bright green eyes, while Judith leaned towards a quiet, gentle gray kitten. They spent time with each, watching how they moved and interacted, and Hannah felt a special connection with the tabby, who seemed equally drawn to her.

Judith and Hannah shared a quiet conversation about what kind of kitten they were looking for. Hannah spoke of her dreams of playing with the kitten in the garden and having a new friend to cuddle with at bedtime. The tabby cat would be perfect.

In the following days, they named their new family member "Lucky" for the good fortune they had found in his playful presence. Hannah and Lucky became inseparable. They played in the garden, cuddled up for story time, and played together. Their home was filled with warmth and laughter.

Hannah and her grandmother had shown the magical moments that come from opening your heart to a new, purring friend.

THE END

The Cat Appointment -
Jamie Stonebridge, Rachel Horon

The Senior Center Cat
The Jazz Emporium's Cat, The Dance Partner
The Cat and the Reading Club
Maine Cat Adventures
The Garden Companion, The Cat Café
Choosing Lucky
- Sam Suncroft

Set in 20 pt EB Garamond
seniorality.com